Table of Contents:

Chapter 1:

The Origins of Yoga

Yoga originated in ancient India over 5,000 years ago and is deeply rooted in spirituality and philosophy. The word "yoga" comes from the Sanskrit word "yuj," which means to unite or join, symbolizing the connection between mind, body, and spirit. Yoga boosts mental wellbeing by focusing on breathing,strength, and flexibility. Yoga was first mentioned in ancient sacred text called "Rig Veda".

Chapter 2:

Understanding the Different Styles of Yoga

There are various styles of yoga, each with its own emphasis and approach. Hatha yoga focuses on physical postures and breath control, while Vinyasa flows between poses with breath synchronization. Ashtanga is a more structured and intense practice, while Kundalini aims to awaken energy within the body. Let's dive into more detail about some popular types of yoga practices, each with its unique focus and benefits:

Hatha Yoga:

Hatha yoga is one of the most widely practiced forms and serves as a foundation for many other styles. It emphasizes physical postures (asanas) and breath control (pranayama). Hatha aims to balance the body and mind, making it an excellent choice for beginners. This style often includes static poses held for a few breaths, allowing practitioners to focus on alignment and relaxation.

Vinyasa Yoga:

Vinyasa is a dynamic and flowing style that synchronizes breath with movement. It involves transitioning smoothly from one pose to another, creating a dance-like sequence. This continuous flow of movements builds strength, flexibility, and cardiovascular endurance while promoting mindfulness. Vinyasa allows for creativity in sequencing, so each class can be unique and engaging.

Ashtanga Yoga:

Ashtanga is a rigorous and structured practice that follows a predefined sequence of postures. It comprises Primary Series, Intermediate Series, and Advanced Series. Practitioners progress through the series as they master each pose. Ashtanga is physically demanding, promoting strength, flexibility, and discipline. It requires commitment and regular practice.

Iyengar Yoga:

Iyengar yoga emphasizes precision and alignment in poses. It uses various props, such as blocks, straps, and bolsters, to support and modify poses for individual needs. This style focuses on detail, helping practitioners achieve proper body alignment and reducing the risk of injury. Iyengar is suitable for all levels and often incorporates longer holds to deepen the experience.

Bikram Yoga (Hot Yoga):

Bikram yoga is practiced in a heated room, typically set at around 105°F (40°C), with high humidity. It follows a fixed sequence of 26 poses and two breathing exercises. The heat is believed to increase flexibility, promote detoxification, and challenge practitioners physically and mentally. However, some caution is advised, especially for individuals with certain medical conditions or heat sensitivity.

Kundalini Yoga:

Kundalini yoga focuses on awakening the dormant energy (kundalini) within the body through dynamic movements, breathwork, and chanting. It aims to balance the chakras and cultivate spiritual awareness. Kundalini classes often include mantra chanting, meditation, and rapid breathwork (pranayama) exercises known as "kriyas."

Yin Yoga:

Yin yoga is a slow-paced and passive practice that targets the connective tissues, such as ligaments and fascia, rather than the muscles. Poses are held for an extended duration, typically 3-5 minutes, allowing for deep stretching and releasing tension. Yin yoga enhances flexibility, joint mobility, and mindfulness, making it a perfect complement to more active practices.

Restorative Yoga:

Restorative yoga is a deeply relaxing practice that uses props to support the body in gentle postures. It is designed to promote relaxation, stress reduction, and healing. Restorative poses are held for an extended time, allowing the nervous system to shift into the parasympathetic mode, known as the "rest and digest" state.

Each type of yoga offers unique benefits, and exploring different styles can enhance your overall yoga experience. Finding the style that resonates with you the most is essential for building a sustainable and enjoyable practice. Remember that all yoga practices emphasize self-awareness, self-compassion, and mindfulness, making it a journey of self-discovery and growth.

Chapter 3:

The Benefits of Yoga

Yoga offers a myriad of benefits for both physical and mental health. Regular practice can improve flexibility, strength, balance, and posture. It also helps reduce stress, anxiety, and depression while promoting mindfulness and inner peace. Yoga offers a wide range of benefits for mental, physical, and spiritual well-being.

Mental Benefits of Yoga:

 Yoga incorporates breathing techniques and meditation, which help activate the parasympathetic nervous system, leading to a relaxation response. This reduces the production of stress hormones like cortisol, alleviating stress and promoting a sense of calm.

Practicing yoga encourages mindfulness and concentration. The act of focusing on breath and body alignment during poses helps clear the mind and enhance mental clarity.

Regular yoga practice can improve emotional resilience and help manage mood swings. It cultivates self-awareness, allowing practitioners to recognize and respond to emotions in a more balanced way.

Yoga has been shown to reduce symptoms of anxiety and depression by promoting the release of mood-regulating neurotransmitters like serotonin. It provides a sense of empowerment and control over one's emotions.

The combination of physical movement, breathwork, and meditation can enhance cognitive function, including memory, attention, and problem-solving abilities.

Physical Benefits of Yoga:

Yoga involves a variety of stretching exercises that improve flexibility and range of motion in joints and muscles. This can reduce the risk of injuries and enhance overall mobility.

Many yoga poses engage and strengthen various muscle groups, contributing to better posture, body alignment, and overall strength.

Balancing poses in yoga challenge the body's equilibrium, helping to enhance balance and coordination.

Some dynamic styles of yoga, like Vinyasa, can provide a cardiovascular workout, increasing heart rate and improving circulation.

The controlled movements and alignment-focused nature of yoga are gentle on joints, making it suitable for people with arthritis or joint issues.

Spiritual Benefits of Yoga:

Yoga encourages introspection and self-awareness, allowing individuals to explore their inner thoughts and emotions, leading to self-discovery and personal growth.

For many practitioners, yoga serves as a spiritual practice that connects them to a higher power, the universe, or a deeper sense of purpose and meaning in life.

Yoga philosophy often emphasizes the importance of compassion and gratitude, fostering a sense of interconnectedness with all living beings.

Regular practice of yoga and meditation can lead to a profound sense of inner peace, tranquility, and contentment.

Yoga's holistic approach aims to unify the mind, body, and spirit, creating a harmonious and balanced sense of being.

Regular practice and dedication are key to experiencing the full range of advantages that yoga has to offer mentally, physically, and spiritually. As with any physical or spiritual practice, it is essential to approach yoga with an open mind and respect for personal limitations.

Chapter 4:

Anatomy and Physiology in Yoga

Understanding anatomy is crucial in practicing yoga safely and effectively. It involves learning about muscles, bones, and joints, as well as the physiological responses of the body during different poses and movements. The practice of yoga involves a profound understanding of human anatomy and physiology to ensure safe and effective execution of poses (asanas) and breathwork (pranayama).

Yoga engages various muscle groups, promoting strength, flexibility, and balance. Muscles work in pairs, contracting and relaxing to allow movement. For instance, in a standing forward fold (Uttanasana), the hamstrings lengthen while the quadriceps contract to support the movement.

The skeletal system provides the framework for yoga postures. Understanding bones and their articulations is crucial for alignment. For example, in Warrior II (Virabhadrasana II), the knee aligns with the ankle, ensuring proper stability and joint safety.

Yoga poses involve different types of joints, such as hinge joints (knees and elbows) and ball-and-socket joints (hips and shoulders). Proper alignment protects these joints from excessive stress during practice.

The spine is essential in yoga, as many poses involve spinal flexion, extension, lateral bending, and rotation. Maintaining a neutral spine is crucial to avoid injury and maintain proper posture.

Pranayama (breath control) is a key component of yoga. Breathing deeply and mindfully enhances lung capacity, oxygenates the body, and calms the nervous system. Understanding the mechanics of breathing aids in breathwork practices.

Yoga influences the autonomic nervous system, which controls involuntary bodily functions. The parasympathetic nervous system is activated during relaxation and meditation, promoting rest and recovery, while the sympathetic nervous system responds to stress and triggers the "fight-or-flight" response.

Dynamic styles of yoga can increase heart rate and circulation, promoting cardiovascular health. Asanas that involve inversions, like headstand (Sirsasana), can facilitate venous return and improve blood flow to the heart.

Certain yoga practices, like shoulderstand (Sarvangasana), stimulate the thyroid gland, which plays a vital role in metabolism and energy regulation. Yoga's stress-reducing benefits also influence hormone balance.

Yoga postures, especially in Yin and Restorative styles, target fascia and connective tissues. These long-held stretches can help release tension, improve joint mobility, and increase flexibility.

The mind-body connection is a fundamental aspect of yoga. Yoga practices encourage self-awareness, which can influence mental and emotional states. Mindfulness techniques in yoga meditation can promote mental clarity and reduce stress.

Understanding the anatomy and physiology of yoga enables practitioners to adapt poses to their unique bodies and avoid potential injuries. Proper alignment, breathwork, and an appreciation for the intricacies of the human body are essential for a safe and rewarding yoga practice. Furthermore, a deeper understanding of the physiological effects of yoga contributes to its therapeutic and transformative benefits on physical, mental, and emotional levels. 🧘🌿

Chapter 5:

The Art of Breathwork (Pranayama)

Breathing techniques, or pranayama, play a significant role in yoga. Proper breath control can enhance concentration, calm the mind, and improve overall respiratory health. Breathwork, known as "pranayama" in yoga, is a fundamental aspect of the practice that involves conscious control and regulation of the breath. Prana refers to the life force or vital energy, and yama means control or expansion. Pranayama techniques offer numerous physical, mental, and emotional benefits. Let's explore the art of breathwork in full detail:

The first step in pranayama is cultivating breath awareness. It involves observing the natural rhythm of the breath without attempting to control it. By bringing attention to the breath, practitioners develop mindfulness and a deeper connection with their internal state.

Also known as "three-part breath," this technique involves deepening the breath by expanding the belly, ribcage, and upper chest. Diaphragmatic breathing engages the full capacity of the lungs, enhancing oxygen intake and calming the nervous system.

Ujjayi breath is often referred to as "victorious breath" or "ocean breath." It involves gently contracting the back of the throat during both inhalation and exhalation, creating a soft hissing or ocean-like sound. Ujjayi breath helps focus the mind, regulates the breath, and generates internal heat during more vigorous yoga practices.

Nadi Shodhana is a balancing pranayama technique that helps harmonize the left and right energy channels (nadis) in the body. By alternating the breath between the left and right nostrils, practitioners can promote a sense of balance, mental clarity, and stress reduction.

Kapalabhati is a cleansing and energizing breathwork technique that involves forceful exhalations and passive inhalations. It helps clear the respiratory passages, invigorates the body, and stimulates digestion.

Bhramari pranayama involves producing a gentle humming sound during exhalation, similar to the sound of a bee. This technique has a calming effect on the mind and nervous system, making it beneficial for stress reduction and anxiety relief.

Sheetali involves inhaling through the rolled tongue or pursed lips to create a cooling sensation. This pranayama helps reduce body temperature, soothes the mind, and calms the nervous system.

Sama Vritti is a simple breathwork technique where the duration of inhalation matches the duration of exhalation. It promotes a state of balance and relaxation and can be helpful for enhancing focus during meditation.

The art of breathwork in yoga is a powerful tool for managing physical and mental states. By incorporating various pranayama techniques into their practice, individuals can enhance their yoga experience, cultivate mindfulness, reduce stress, and improve overall well-being. Regular and consistent pranayama practice allows practitioners to develop a deeper connection with their breath and harness the transformative power of controlled breathing in various aspects of their lives.

Chapter 6:

Mastering the Fundamental Poses

Yoga poses, or asanas, form the core of any yoga practice. This chapter will explore essential poses, including downward-facing dog, warrior series, and child's pose, along with their alignment and benefits.
Mastering the fundamental poses of yoga requires patience, practice, and attention to detail. These poses serve as the foundation for more advanced postures and are essential for building strength, flexibility, and body awareness. Let's explore the key details and alignment cues for some of the fundamental yoga poses:

1. Mountain Pose (Tadasana):

- Stand with feet hip-width apart, toes pointing forward, and weight evenly distributed.
- Engage the thighs, draw the belly in, and lift the chest.
- Relax the shoulders away from the ears and lengthen the neck.
- Gaze straight ahead and breathe deeply.

2. Downward-Facing Dog (Adho Mukha Svanasana):

- Start in a tabletop position with hands shoulder-width apart and knees hip-width apart.
- Press into the palms, lift the knees off the mat, and straighten the legs.
- Hips move up and back, forming an inverted "V" shape.
- Heels may or may not touch the mat; focus on lengthening the spine and engaging the core.

3. Plank Pose:

- From a push-up position, align the shoulders directly over the wrists.
- Engage the core, quads, and glutes to form a straight line from head to heels.
- Avoid sinking the hips or arching the back.

4. Warrior I (Virabhadrasana I):

- Step one foot forward into a lunge position, with the knee directly over the ankle.
- Back foot is at a 45-degree angle with the heel rooted to the mat.
- Square the hips and lift the torso, reaching the arms overhead with palms facing each other.
- Gaze forward or upward, and engage the core for stability.

5. Warrior II (Virabhadrasana II):

- From Warrior I, open the hips and arms out to the sides.
- Front foot points forward, and back foot maintains the 45-degree angle.
- Arms extend parallel to the floor, shoulders relaxed, and gaze over the front middle finger.
- Keep the front knee bent at a 90-degree angle, ensuring it aligns with the ankle.

6. Triangle Pose (Trikonasana):

- Step the feet wide apart, with the front foot pointing forward and the back foot at a 90-degree angle.
- Reach the front arm forward, hinging at the hip, and place the hand on the shin, ankle, or floor.
- The other arm extends upward, creating a straight line from fingertips to fingertips.
- Gaze up toward the top hand or downward if more comfortable for the neck.

7. Child's Pose (Balasana):

- Kneel on the mat with big toes touching and knees wide apart.

- Sit back on the heels and fold the torso forward, reaching the arms out in front or alongside the body.
- Rest the forehead on the mat and breathe deeply into the back and sides of the body.

8. Corpse Pose (Savasana):

- Lie flat on the mat with legs extended and arms by the sides, palms facing up.
- Close the eyes and relax the entire body, releasing any tension.
- Focus on the breath and remain still for a few minutes, allowing the body and mind to settle.

Mastering these fundamental yoga poses involves paying attention to proper alignment, engaging the right muscles, and using the breath to deepen the experience.

Chapter 7:

Sun Salutations - The Heart of Yoga

Sun salutations are dynamic sequences that warm up the body and link breath with movement. They are an integral part of many yoga practices and offer a great full-body workout. Sun Salutations, also known as Surya Namaskar, are a series of flowing yoga poses traditionally practiced at the beginning of a yoga session to warm up the body and connect with the breath. The sequence consists of several postures that stretch, strengthen, and energize different parts of the body. Let's explore the detailed steps of the Sun Salutations:

There are different variations of Sun Salutations, and I'll describe the classical version, Surya Namaskar A, commonly practiced in Hatha and Vinyasa yoga styles:

1. Mountain Pose (Tadasana):

   - Stand tall with feet together or hip-width apart, grounding into the mat.
   - Bring hands together at the heart center (Anjali Mudra).
   - Take a few deep breaths to center and prepare for the flow.

2. Upward Salute (Urdhva Hastasana):

   - Inhale, extend the arms overhead, palms facing each other.
   - Gently arch the back, lifting the chest, and lengthening the spine.
   - Keep the shoulders relaxed away from the ears.

3. Forward Fold (Uttanasana):

   - Exhale, hinge at the hips, and fold forward, reaching for the toes or shins.

- Keep the spine long and the legs as straight as comfortable (bend the knees if needed).
- Relax the neck and breathe deeply into the back body.

4. Halfway Lift (Ardha Uttanasana):

   - Inhale, lengthen the spine forward, keeping the back flat.
   - Place hands on shins or fingertips on the mat, gazing slightly forward.

5. Plank Pose:

   - Exhale, step or jump both feet back into a push-up position.
   - Align the shoulders over the wrists and engage the core and legs.
   - Keep the body in a straight line from head to heels.

6. Low Plank (Chaturanga Dandasana):

   - As you lower down, keep the elbows close to the body.
   - Hover the body a few inches above the mat, engaging the triceps.

7. Upward-Facing Dog (Urdhva Mukha Svanasana):

   - Inhale, roll over the toes, and lift the chest upward.
   - Press the palms into the mat, straightening the arms.
   - The tops of the feet and thighs remain on the mat.

8. Downward-Facing Dog (Adho Mukha Svanasana):

   - Exhale, lift the hips up and back into an inverted "V" shape.
   - Press the palms firmly into the mat, spreading the fingers wide.
   - Heels aim toward the floor, and the head is relaxed between the arms.

9. Halfway Lift (Ardha Uttanasana):

   - Inhale, look forward, and step or hop to the top of the mat.
   - Lengthen the spine as in the previous halfway lift.

10. Forward Fold (Uttanasana):

   - Exhale, fold forward again, deepening the stretch.

11. Upward Salute (Urdhva Hastasana):

   - Inhale, sweep the arms overhead, returning to the upward salute.

12. Mountain Pose (Tadasana):

   - Exhale, bring the hands back to the heart center, completing one full round of Sun Salutation.

To continue with another round, repeat the steps from Upward Salute (step 2) to Mountain Pose (step 12). Traditionally, Sun Salutations are performed in sets of 5 or 12 rounds, but you can adjust the number according to your time and energy level.

Sun Salutations offer a full-body workout, combining strength, flexibility, and breathwork. They are an excellent way to energize the body, warm up the muscles, and prepare for a more extended yoga practice or meditation session. Practice Sun Salutations regularly, and you'll experience increased vitality, improved flexibility, and a deeper connection to your breath and body.

Chapter 8:

Yoga Props and Their Uses

Props like blocks, straps, and bolsters are valuable tools that assist practitioners in achieving proper alignment and making yoga accessible to everyone, regardless of their flexibility or experience.
Yoga props are valuable tools that can enhance your yoga practice by providing support, stability, and accessibility in various poses. They are especially helpful for beginners, individuals with physical limitations, or those seeking to deepen their practice. Here's a brief overview of common yoga props and how to use them:

1. Yoga Blocks:

   - Blocks are typically made of foam, cork, or wood and come in various sizes.
   - They provide height and support to help with proper alignment in standing, seated, and balancing poses.
   - Use them to bring the floor closer to you in forward folds or to modify challenging poses like Triangle Pose, placing a block under your hand or supporting your lower hand on a block.

2. Yoga Straps:

   - Straps are long, flexible bands made of cotton or nylon with a buckle or D-ring for adjustments.
   - They assist in stretching and reaching in poses where flexibility is limited, such as seated forward bends or binding poses.
   - Wrap the strap around your feet in seated forward bends to reach your hands toward your toes, or use it to hold your hands in Gomukhasana (Cow Face Pose) when you cannot reach them together behind your back.

3. Yoga Bolsters:

   - Bolsters are firm, cylindrical or rectangular cushions often filled with cotton or foam.
   - They provide support and comfort in restorative and yin yoga poses, allowing you to relax and hold poses for an extended duration.
   - Use a bolster under your knees in Savasana (Corpse Pose) for added relaxation, or place it under your back in a supported bridge pose to open the chest.

4. Yoga Blankets:

   - Yoga blankets are versatile and can be folded or rolled to provide cushioning or support.
   - They offer padding under knees, hips, or shoulders in various poses like Camel Pose or Shoulderstand.
   - Use a rolled-up blanket to support the neck in Fish Pose or sit on a folded blanket to elevate the hips in seated poses.

5. Yoga Wheels:

   - Yoga wheels are circular props made of foam or wood, designed to support backbends, hip openers, and shoulder stretches.
   - They can help deepen stretches and improve flexibility in poses like Bridge Pose or Wheel Pose.
   - Gently roll the back over the wheel to massage and release tension in the spine.

6. Meditation Cushions:

   - Meditation cushions, like zafus or zabutons, provide comfort and support during seated meditation.
   - They elevate the hips, allowing for a more comfortable and aligned sitting position, reducing strain on the knees and back.

Using yoga props can make poses more accessible and safer, helping you maintain proper alignment and prevent injuries. Experiment with different props to find what works best for your body and practice. As you progress, you may find that your need for props changes, and you can gradually incorporate more challenging variations without them. Remember, yoga props are there to assist and support you on your journey to a fulfilling and transformative yoga practice.

Chapter 9:

Practicing Meditation and Mindfulness

Yoga isn't just about physical postures; meditation and mindfulness are integral components. This chapter will explore various meditation techniques and their positive effects on mental well-being.

Meditation and mindfulness are essential components of yoga that cultivate inner awareness, presence, and mental clarity. They play a significant role in calming the mind, reducing stress, and promoting overall well-being.

Meditation:

Meditation is a technique used to focus and quiet the mind, promoting a state of mental clarity and emotional calmness. There are various meditation techniques, but the core principles remain consistent:

1. Mindful Breathing (Anapanasati):

  - One of the most common meditation techniques, it involves focusing attention on the breath.
  - Sit comfortably and observe the natural rhythm of your breath, feeling the inhalation and exhalation.
  - When the mind wanders, gently bring the focus back to the breath without judgment.

2. Loving-Kindness Meditation (Metta):

  - Metta meditation is a practice of cultivating compassion and love for oneself and others.
  - Start by sending well-wishes to yourself, then gradually extend those wishes to loved ones, acquaintances, and even challenging individuals.
  - This practice fosters feelings of connection and empathy, promoting emotional well-being.

3. Body Scan Meditation:

   - In body scan meditation, attention is directed systematically through different parts of the
body, cultivating body awareness and relaxation.
   - Start at the top of the head and progressively move down to the toes, observing sensations
without attachment or aversion.

4. Transcendental Meditation (TM):

   - TM is a technique where practitioners use a specific mantra, a word or sound, to achieve a
state of deep relaxation and self-awareness.
   - This practice involves repeating the mantra silently to oneself and effortlessly returning to it
when thoughts arise.

Mindfulness:

Mindfulness is the practice of bringing full attention and awareness to the present moment
without judgment. It involves acknowledging thoughts, emotions, and sensations as they arise,
observing them without attachment or resistance. Mindfulness is often incorporated into daily
activities and can be applied in various ways:

1. Mindful Eating:

   - Paying attention to the taste, texture, and smell of food while eating mindfully.
   - Avoiding distractions and savoring each bite, fully experiencing the nourishment.

2. Mindful Walking:

   - Engaging fully in the act of walking, observing the movement of the body, and feeling the
ground beneath the feet.
   - Letting go of distractions and focusing solely on the present moment.

3. Mindful Listening:

   - Giving undivided attention when someone is speaking, without interrupting or thinking of a
response.
   - Being fully present and open to understanding the speaker's words and emotions.

4. Mindful Daily Activities:

- Engaging with routine tasks like washing dishes, brushing teeth, or driving with full attention and without rushing through them.

The practice of meditation and mindfulness in yoga fosters a sense of presence and self-awareness. Regular practice can lead to reduced stress, improved focus, emotional regulation, and a greater sense of inner peace. It's essential to approach these practices with patience and compassion, as meditation and mindfulness are skills that develop over time with consistent practice. Whether seated on a cushion or being fully present in everyday activities, cultivating these practices enhances the overall quality of life and brings a deeper connection to oneself and the world.

Chapter 10:

Yoga Philosophy and Ethical Principles

Yoga philosophy encompasses the Yamas and Niyamas, ethical guidelines that encourage personal growth, compassion, and self-awareness.

Chapter 11:

Preparing for Advanced Yoga Poses

Advanced yoga poses require patience, dedication, and a deep understanding of foundational poses. Proper preparation and guidance are essential to avoid injuries.

Chapter 12:

Yoga for Special Populations

Yoga can be adapted to suit various individuals, including seniors, pregnant women, and people with physical limitations. This chapter will delve into modifications and considerations for specific populations.

Chapter 13:

The Chakras and Energy Centers

The ancient yogic system recognizes seven chakras, or energy centers, located along the spine. Understanding these energy points can aid in balancing the body and mind.
Chakras are energy centers within the subtle body of yoga and other spiritual systems. They are believed to be spinning wheels or vortexes of energy that regulate the flow of life force or prana throughout the body. Each chakra is associated with specific physical, emotional, and spiritual aspects. Understanding and balancing the chakras can lead to a more harmonious and balanced state of being.

1. Root Chakra (Muladhara):

- Location: Base of the spine, at the perineum.
- Element: Earth.
- Color: Red.
- Physical Associations: Legs, feet, bones, lower back, adrenal glands.
- Emotional Associations: Survival instincts, security, stability, grounding.
- Balanced Characteristics: Feeling safe, secure, and grounded. Strong sense of stability and connection to the physical world.

2. Sacral Chakra (Svadhisthana):

- Location: Below the navel, near the sacrum.
- Element: Water.
- Color: Orange.
- Physical Associations: Reproductive organs, lower abdomen, hips, kidneys.
- Emotional Associations: Creativity, sensuality, emotional expression, pleasure.
- Balanced Characteristics: Embracing creativity, having healthy emotional boundaries, and experiencing pleasure and intimacy.

3. Solar Plexus Chakra (Manipura):

- Location: Above the navel, at the solar plexus.
- Element: Fire.
- Color: Yellow.
- Physical Associations: Digestive system, abdomen, liver, pancreas.
- Emotional Associations: Self-confidence, personal power, willpower, self-esteem.
- Balanced Characteristics: Feeling confident, having a strong sense of personal power, and being self-motivated.

4. Heart Chakra (Anahata):

- Location: Center of the chest, near the heart.
- Element: Air.

- Color: Green (also associated with pink).
- Physical Associations: Heart, lungs, chest, circulatory system.
- Emotional Associations: Love, compassion, forgiveness, empathy.
- Balanced Characteristics: Feeling love for oneself and others, fostering compassion, and having healthy relationships.

5. Throat Chakra (Vishuddha):

- Location: Throat region.
- Element: Ether or Sound.
- Color: Blue (also associated with turquoise).
- Physical Associations: Throat, neck, thyroid gland.
- Emotional Associations: Communication, self-expression, authenticity.
- Balanced Characteristics: Being able to express oneself clearly and authentically, speaking one's truth with compassion.

6. Third Eye Chakra (Ajna):

- Location: Between the eyebrows, slightly above.
- Element: Light.
- Color: Indigo (dark blue).
- Physical Associations: Pituitary gland, brain, eyes.
- Emotional Associations: Intuition, imagination, inner wisdom.
- Balanced Characteristics: Heightened intuition, clarity of thought, and a strong connection to inner guidance.

7. Crown Chakra (Sahasrara):

- Location: Top of the head.
- Element: Consciousness.
- Color: Violet or white.
- Physical Associations: Pineal gland, brain.
- Emotional Associations: Spiritual connection, universal consciousness, enlightenment.
- Balanced Characteristics: Feeling connected to the divine and experiencing a sense of spiritual unity.

The balanced functioning of all seven chakras is believed to promote physical, emotional, and spiritual well-being. When a chakra is blocked or imbalanced, it can lead to physical ailments, emotional disturbances, and a sense of disconnection. Various practices, such as yoga, meditation, breathwork, and energy healing, can help to unblock and balance the chakras, supporting a more integrated and holistic state of being.

Chapter 14:

Yoga for Stress Relief and Relaxation

Yoga's emphasis on deep breathing and mindfulness techniques makes it an effective tool for managing stress and promoting relaxation.
Yoga Is a powerful tool for stress relief and relaxation, offering various practices that promote physical, mental, and emotional well-being. Here are some of the key aspects of how yoga helps alleviate stress and induces relaxation:

1. Physical Benefits:

   - Relaxation Response: The practice of yoga activates the parasympathetic nervous system, triggering the body's relaxation response. This counters the "fight-or-flight" stress response, leading to a calmer state of being.
   - Reduced Muscle Tension: Yoga poses involve stretching and releasing muscle tension, which helps reduce physical stress stored in the body.
   - **Improved Sleep:** Regular yoga practice can enhance sleep quality by calming the mind and reducing stress hormones that can interfere with sleep.

2. Breathwork (Pranayama):

   - Deep Breathing: Breathing exercises in yoga, such as diaphragmatic breathing and Ujjayi breath, help slow down the breath, relax the nervous system, and reduce anxiety.
   - Alternate Nostril Breathing: Nadi Shodhana pranayama balances the left and right brain hemispheres, promoting mental clarity and emotional balance.

3. Mindfulness and Meditation:

   - Present Moment Awareness: Mindfulness practices in yoga help bring awareness to the present moment, reducing the tendency to ruminate on past events or worry about the future.
   - Stress Reduction: Meditation techniques, like loving-kindness meditation or body scan meditation, reduce stress by promoting a sense of inner calm and emotional regulation.

4. Yoga Nidra (Yogic Sleep):

   - Yoga Nidra is a guided meditation and relaxation practice that induces a state of deep relaxation, equivalent to a few hours of restful sleep. It helps alleviate physical, mental, and emotional stress.

5. Restorative Yoga:

   - Restorative yoga uses props and supportive postures to provide deep relaxation and release tension. It promotes the activation of the parasympathetic nervous system, leading to profound relaxation.

6. Mind-Body Connection:
   - Yoga encourages a strong mind-body connection, promoting self-awareness and self-compassion. This helps individuals recognize and address stress triggers more effectively.

7. Emotional Regulation:

   - Yoga fosters emotional regulation, allowing practitioners to acknowledge and process emotions in a healthy way, reducing stress and anxiety.

8. Community and Support:

   - Practicing yoga in a supportive community or with a qualified teacher can create a sense of connection and belonging, reducing feelings of isolation and stress.

9. Sensory Withdrawal (Pratyahara):

   - Pratyahara, the withdrawal of the senses, is a preparatory practice for meditation. By turning attention inward, it helps detach from external stimuli and promotes relaxation.

10. Hormonal Balance:

   - Yoga's stress-relieving effects can help balance hormone levels, reducing the production of stress hormones like cortisol and promoting a sense of well-being.

Consistent yoga practice offers a holistic approach to stress relief and relaxation. Integrating various aspects of yoga, including physical postures, breathwork, meditation, and mindfulness, helps individuals manage stress more effectively and develop coping mechanisms for life's challenges. By making yoga a regular part of your routine, you can cultivate a calmer mind, a relaxed body, and an overall sense of balance and well-being.

Chapter 15:

Partner and Acro Yoga

Partner and Acro yoga foster trust, communication, and connection with others. These practices involve two or more individuals working together in various poses and sequences.
Partner Yoga and Acro Yoga are two fun and interactive styles of yoga that involve practicing yoga poses and flows with a partner or in a group. Both styles emphasize trust, communication, and connection between participants. Let's explore each style in full detail:

1. Partner Yoga:

Partner Yoga involves practicing yoga postures and flows with a partner. It allows participants to deepen stretches, improve balance, and explore poses that might be challenging individually. Partner Yoga fosters communication, cooperation, and a sense of support.

Benefits of Partner Yoga:

- Enhanced Stretching: Partners can assist each other in lengthening muscles and reaching deeper stretches.
- Increased Balance and Stability: Practicing poses together can provide additional support and stability, allowing participants to explore more advanced postures.
- Building Trust and Connection: Partner Yoga involves physical touch and requires trust and communication between partners, creating a deeper sense of connection and intimacy.
- Shared Experience: Partner Yoga allows participants to share the practice, creating a bonding experience and sense of togetherness.

2. Acro Yoga:

Acro Yoga combines yoga, acrobatics, and Thai massage elements to create a dynamic and playful practice. It involves three main roles: the base, the flyer, and the spotter. The base supports the flyer in elevated poses, while the spotter ensures safety and provides guidance.

Benefits of Acro Yoga:

- Strength and Conditioning: Acro Yoga builds strength in the core, arms, and legs as participants support and lift each other.
- Trust and Communication: Practicing Acro poses requires clear communication and trust between the base and flyer, fostering strong connections.
- Playfulness and Joy: Acro Yoga encourages participants to explore their playful side and experience the joy of flying and being lifted.
- Therapeutic Element: Acro Yoga often involves therapeutic flying and Thai massage techniques, promoting relaxation and stress relief.

Safety Considerations:

Both Partner Yoga and Acro Yoga are generally safe when practiced mindfully and with proper communication. Here are some safety tips:
- Work with a partner you trust and establish clear communication signals.
- Start with simple poses and progress gradually to more advanced ones.
- Always warm up the body before attempting any acrobatic moves.
- Use proper spotting techniques and have a spotter when practicing Acro poses.
- Be mindful of each other's physical limitations and comfort levels.

Partner Yoga and Acro Yoga offer unique and enjoyable ways to share the yoga practice with others, fostering trust, connection, and playfulness. Whether you prefer the grounded and supportive nature of Partner Yoga or the dynamic and acrobatic elements of Acro Yoga, both styles provide an opportunity to deepen your yoga practice and create meaningful connections with others. Remember to practice with safety and respect for each other's boundaries, and most importantly, have fun!

Chapter 16:

The Yoga Lifestyle

Beyond the mat, the yoga lifestyle includes conscious eating, eco-friendly choices, and living with intention and gratitude. Yoga lifestyle and healthy eating are integral components of a holistic yoga practice that extends beyond the physical postures on the mat. Embracing a yoga lifestyle involves adopting mindful habits, nurturing the body and mind, and fostering a sense of balance and well-being. Let's explore each aspect in full detail:

1. Yoga Lifestyle:

- Mindfulness: A yoga lifestyle emphasizes living in the present moment, cultivating awareness, and being mindful of thoughts, actions, and emotions.
- Simplicity: Simplifying life by decluttering physical possessions and reducing unnecessary distractions helps create a calmer and more focused mind.
- Gratitude: Practicing gratitude fosters a positive outlook and appreciation for life's blessings, promoting contentment and joy.
- Compassion: Embracing compassion toward oneself and others cultivates empathy, kindness, and a deeper sense of connection.
- Self-Care: Prioritizing self-care through practices like yoga, meditation, spending time in nature, or engaging in creative activities nourishes the mind, body, and soul.
- Connection with Nature: Spending time in nature and cultivating an appreciation for the environment enhances the sense of interconnectedness and environmental consciousness.

2. Eating Healthy in Yoga:

- Plant-Based Diet: Many yogis follow a plant-based or vegetarian diet, as it aligns with the principle of ahimsa (non-harming) and promotes ethical eating.
- Whole Foods: Choosing whole, unprocessed foods such as fruits, vegetables, grains, nuts, and seeds provides essential nutrients and supports overall well-being.
- Mindful Eating: Being present and fully engaged in the eating process, savoring flavors, and eating slowly helps prevent overeating and fosters better digestion.
- Hydration: Drinking sufficient water throughout the day supports proper bodily functions and maintains hydration.
- Moderation: Practicing moderation in food intake helps maintain a balanced diet and prevents overindulgence or restrictive eating habits.
- Eating with Awareness: Understanding how different foods affect the body and mind empowers individuals to make conscious and nourishing food choices.
- Fasting: Some yogic traditions incorporate occasional fasting as a way to cleanse and purify the body and mind.

3. Cooking with Mindfulness:

- Cooking as a Meditation: Preparing meals with mindfulness, focus, and intention can turn cooking into a meditative and soul-nourishing experience.
- Use of Fresh Ingredients: Opting for fresh, seasonal ingredients maximizes nutritional value and enhances the flavors of dishes.
- Herbs and Spices: Utilizing herbs and spices in cooking not only adds flavor but also offers various health benefits.
- Balanced Meals: Creating well-balanced meals that incorporate a variety of nutrients, colors, and textures supports overall health and vitality.
- Food as Fuel: Viewing food as fuel for the body helps make conscious choices that promote energy and well-being.

Adopting a yoga lifestyle and eating healthily go hand in hand to support physical, mental, and spiritual well-being. Embracing mindfulness, simplicity, compassion, and gratitude fosters a deeper connection to oneself and the world. A balanced and nourishing diet complements the physical practice of yoga and contributes to a harmonious and holistic approach to life. Remember that each person's journey is unique, and finding what works best for you is essential in creating a sustainable and fulfilling yoga lifestyle.

Chapter 17:

Yoga and Scientific Research

Explore the growing body of scientific research supporting the physical and mental benefits of yoga, from reducing inflammation to enhancing brain function. Scientific research on yoga has grown significantly over the years, and numerous studies have explored its effects on physical, mental, and emotional well-being. Here are some key findings from scientific research on yoga:

Physical Benefits:

- Flexibility: Regular yoga practice improves flexibility by stretching and lengthening muscles, as shown in studies published in the Journal of Physical Therapy Science and the International Journal of Yoga Therapy.
- Strength: Yoga poses, especially those involving bodyweight resistance, can increase muscle strength and endurance, according to research published in the International Journal of Yoga.
- Balance: A systematic review published in the Journal of Aging Research suggests that yoga practice enhances balance and reduces the risk of falls, especially in older adults.
- Cardiovascular Health: Several studies, including research published in the European Journal of Preventive Cardiology, indicate that yoga can reduce blood pressure, cholesterol levels, and other cardiovascular risk factors.

Mental and Emotional Benefits:

- Stress Reduction: Numerous studies, including one published in the Journal of Alternative and Complementary Medicine, show that yoga can lower cortisol levels (stress hormone) and reduce perceived stress and anxiety.
- Depression and Mood: Research published in the Journal of Psychiatric Practice suggests that yoga may complement conventional treatments for depression and improve mood.
- Cognition and Brain Health: Preliminary research, such as a study published in the Journal of Alzheimer's Disease, indicates that yoga may have positive effects on cognitive function and brain health.
- Sleep Quality: A review published in the journal Sleep Science shows that yoga practice can improve sleep quality and reduce insomnia symptoms.

Pain Management:

- Chronic Pain: Studies, including research published in JAMA Internal Medicine, suggest that yoga can help manage chronic pain conditions, such as low back pain, arthritis, and fibromyalgia.
- Headaches and Migraines: Research published in the International Journal of Yoga Therapy indicates that yoga may reduce the frequency and intensity of headaches and migraines.

Immune System Support:

- Research published in the journal Frontiers in Immunology suggests that yoga and meditation practices can positively impact immune system function, potentially boosting overall health and immunity.

Mindfulness and Self-Regulation:

- Brain Changes: Neuroimaging studies, such as those reported in the Journal of Alternative and Complementary Medicine, show that yoga practice can lead to structural and functional changes in the brain associated with improved self-regulation, emotional processing, and attention.

Overall Quality of Life:

- Several studies, such as one published in the journal Cancer, show that yoga can improve overall quality of life and psychological well-being in cancer patients and survivors.

It's important to note that while scientific research on yoga is extensive and promising, there may be variations in study designs, populations, and yoga styles, which can influence results. Additionally, individual responses to yoga can differ, and not everyone may experience the same benefits.

Overall, the scientific evidence strongly supports the numerous positive effects of yoga on physical, mental, and emotional health. As research continues to evolve, yoga's role as a complementary practice for promoting well-being and managing various health conditions becomes increasingly recognized and validated.

Chapter 18:

Yoga Retreats and Traveling for Yoga

Yoga retreats provide an opportunity to immerse oneself in practice while traveling to beautiful destinations. Make sure you do enough research and verify the companies for yoga retreats or traveling to groups.

Chapter 19:

The Future of Yoga

As yoga continues to evolve, this chapter will explore its potential trends and impact on global health and well-being.

Chapter 20:

Embracing Yoga as a Lifelong Journey

Yoga is a lifelong journey of self-discovery and growth. Embracing its principles and practices can lead to profound personal transformation and inner harmony.
Embracing yoga as a lifelong journey and incorporating a routine of yoga can lead to profound physical, mental, and spiritual growth. Yoga is not just a physical exercise; it is a holistic practice that encompasses various aspects of well-being. Here are some factual details on how to embrace yoga as a lifelong journey and establish a regular yoga routine:

Understanding Yoga as a Lifelong Journey:

- Mindset Shift: Embrace yoga as a journey rather than a destination. Recognize that there is always more to learn and explore, both on and off the mat.
- Self-Discovery: Use yoga as a tool for self-discovery and self-awareness. Observe how your practice evolves over time, and be open to new experiences.
- Non-Attachment: Cultivate a sense of non-attachment to expectations and outcomes. Allow your practice to unfold naturally, without judgment or comparison to others.
- Adaptability: Embrace yoga as a lifelong practice that can adapt to different life stages, circumstances, and physical abilities.

Establishing a Yoga Routine:

- Consistency: Commit to a regular yoga practice. Consistency is key to experiencing the benefits of yoga over time.
- Start Small: Begin with a manageable routine that fits into your daily schedule. Even a short daily practice can have a positive impact.
- Set Goals: Set realistic goals for your yoga practice. These could be related to physical progress, increased flexibility, reduced stress, or simply finding more inner peace.
- Variety: Include a variety of yoga styles and practices in your routine, such as Hatha, Vinyasa, Restorative, or Yin Yoga, to keep your practice engaging and well-rounded.
- Listen to Your Body: Pay attention to your body's needs and adjust your practice accordingly. Some days may call for a more gentle practice, while others may invite more dynamic flows.
- Create a Sacred Space: Designate a space for your practice that feels sacred and inviting. This can be a corner of a room, a dedicated yoga studio, or even a quiet outdoor spot.

Integrating Yoga Beyond the Mat:

- Mindful Living: Carry the principles of yoga, such as mindfulness, compassion, and non-violence, into your daily life. Practice being present and mindful in everyday activities.
- Breathwork and Meditation: Incorporate breathwork (pranayama) and meditation into your routine to further deepen your yoga practice and promote mental clarity and relaxation.
- Yoga Philosophy: Study the philosophy of yoga, including the Yoga Sutras, Bhagavad Gita, or other yogic texts, to gain deeper insights into the wisdom and teachings of yoga.
- Yoga Community: Engage with the yoga community by attending workshops, classes, or retreats, or connect with like-minded practitioners to share experiences and support each other.

Self-Compassion and Patience:
- Be Kind to Yourself: Be patient and compassionate with yourself throughout your yoga journey. Progress in yoga is not linear, and it's okay to have ups and downs.
- Celebrate Progress: Celebrate your progress, no matter how small. Acknowledge the growth you experience physically, mentally, and emotionally through your practice.

Remember that yoga is a personal and individual journey. Embrace the process, stay curious, and approach your yoga practice with an open heart and mind. As you cultivate a lifelong relationship with yoga, you'll discover its transformative power in enriching every aspect of your life.

Yoga, with its ancient roots and modern applications, offers a multitude of factual benefits that extend far beyond the physical practice on the mat. Through a holistic approach, yoga enhances physical health by improving flexibility, strength, and balance. Scientific research reveals its positive impact on mental and emotional well-being, reducing stress, anxiety, and depression. With mindfulness and breathwork at its core, yoga fosters self-awareness, leading to greater emotional regulation and inner peace. As a lifelong journey, yoga promotes personal growth and self-discovery, encouraging practitioners to embrace self-compassion and non-attachment. Through its integration into daily life, yoga becomes a powerful tool for mindful living and creating a deeper connection to oneself and others. The practice of yoga offers an empowering and transformative path towards achieving overall well-being and harmonizing mind, body, and spirit.